BORING DIET

Weight Loss Without Hunger, A Path to Healthy Food and Clean Eating

TOM ARMSTRONG

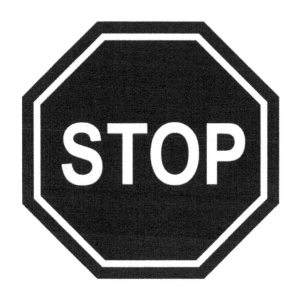

FREE BONUS

Visit BoringDietBook.com to join the email list and receive free access to a bonus video of Tom discussing common questions readers have about *The Boring Diet*.

DISCLAIMER

While best efforts have been made to ensure the accuracy of the information in this book, it is a narrative of the author's personal experience and not a substitute for the medical advice of health care professionals. Before making changes to your diet, please consult a professional.

Copyright © 2020 Tom Armstrong

All Rights Reserved

Table of Contents

Introduction 7

Changing My Family Tree 10

My Moment of Realization... 13

Why We Overeat... 20

The Biochemistry of Food Addiction 25

The Boring Diet 35

   Foods to Definitely Eliminate from Your Environment........38

   Foods to Possibly Eliminate 40

   What You Should Eat...49

   The Heart of the Boring Diet...53

   Suggested Menus 54
      Standard Menu 55
      Scaling the Diet Up or Down...59

   Weekly Schedule 60

   Daily Weighing...61

   How It Works 61

   Summary..62

   That's It?..63

Getting Real About Junk Food 66

Details, Questions, Objections 71

    Nutrition 71

    Breakfast Alternatives 72

    Adherence 75

    Women & Smaller Men 77

    Exercise 79

    The Valley of Fat Loss 82

    What if I'm Already Fit 89

    Artificial & Natural Low Calorie Sweeteners 91

Final Thoughts 95

Introduction

Anyone who was young in the '90s knows about *Seinfeld*. The show famously about nothing created some of the most memorable characters on television. One of those was the Soup Nazi. A grumpy restaurant owner who sold the best soup in the city, the Soup Nazi was famous for ejecting customers from his shop on the smallest of pretenses. If a customer took too long to order or otherwise annoyed him, he would scream, "NO SOUP FOR YOU" and make the customer leave the shop.

I don't remember the first time I was called a "Sugar Nazi" after I changed my relationship with food and eating and purged tempting foods, especially soda, from my home and work environments. When you think about it, it's rather bizarre.

Jerry Seinfeld didn't invent the pop culture use of "Nazi" to describe disciplined enthusiasm, but it's a strange phenomenon how the word Nazi came to signify someone who is overly serious about anything. I think it says something about American culture today that anyone who is serious about something–health, work, grammar–can be nicknamed an XYZ Nazi. Our culture has become so undisciplined that we use a term for our adversary in World War II to jokingly describe strident seriousness in pursuing goals.

Somehow, I don't think this is how the Americans of the 1940s would have seen themselves. Americans are a great people, but we have fallen away from our 20th century peak and into self-indulgence and consumerism. One manifestation of this is the obesity crisis.

We have, to some degree, been tricked into this by the processed food companies, the agricultural lobby, and bad nutrition advice from our own government. We control none of these factors, however. Reformation must begin one individual at a time, by discovering the factors that cause overeating and a determining to change.

In this short book I will describe my journey from the Standard American Diet, and near obesity, to a healthy weight, and more importantly, how I have successfully avoided taking my children down the same road. I will share my best understanding of the science, in the simplest language I can muster.

I am a Christian, so at times, and hopefully not obnoxiously, I will talk about the struggle with weight in spiritual terms. I think everyone can agree that the framework of spirituality has often been useful to humans when trying to balance long-term benefits with short-term pleasure. Even secular folks may find it useful to adopt this framework for this limited purpose.

I also, at times, may use language that can come across as harsh. I know the self-image issues that often come with weight: as a former overweight person, I've experienced them myself. The language I use in places is the same language I use internally to motivate myself. But if you're not in a place right now where tough, uncompromising language is helpful, you won't offend me or anyone else by not reading this book or cutting it short once you read something that hurts you. My psychology might be different than others', and I can only speak from my own experience.

I don't plan to "gift" this book to anyone in particular (a weight loss book might be the least welcome gift ever), so please know I'm not talking to you personally. I'm talking to the reader who is ready to take this journey and ready for some tough love at times to achieve a great result.

I don't recommend taking my advice blindly, but testing it for yourself. I'm not a doctor, just an independent, analytical thinker. I have had some success in business, which helps me sort through complex information amid uncertainty to develop practical plans of action. The doctors don't seem to have the answers either, given the obesity epidemic. I hope what I say makes sense and is useful to you, but test it for yourself, take what's useful, and discard the rest.

Changing My Family Tree

I knew I had accomplished something significant on September 14, 2019. It was about 1:00 p.m., and my older kids had just finished up at a cross-country race in the blistering Southeast Texas heat. There were six of us: myself, my wife, and four daughters ranging in age from eight to fifteen. We were hot, hungry, and about an hour from home. The meet had been in a small town with the typical unhealthy fast-food dining choices. My wife and I decided on Whataburger as our least worst option.

After we ordered—opting out of meal deals, drinking water, and splitting an order of fries among everyone—the good folks at Whataburger delivered our food to the table. As we unwrapped our sandwiches, a couple of my girls looked at me confusedly. Where were they supposed to set their meal? Where were the plates? They had been inside a fast-food restaurant so few times in their lives that they didn't know: the wrapper is the plate.

I looked at my girls and did not resent their joy in experiencing their rare, fast-food meal. They are healthy, skinny, and lanky in the way young people should be, and they could enjoy this occasional treat without guilt because the dose makes the poison. We do not indulge often, and this provides a double benefit. When they do get junk food, they enjoy it more since they haven't built up a tolerance. And when they do enjoy it, there is no guilt because we are not adding to an existing problem. It is a good pleasure because it is experienced in moderation.

Dave Ramsey, the personal finance talk-show host, challenges his listeners to "change their family tree" by being responsible with money. Our experience with food is a direct correspondence to that of money. We must live and eat within our means, and keep the splurges within controlled limits. Otherwise, we end up broke or fat. There is no free lunch, literally or figuratively.

My kids do not have good genetics for this, depending on how you define "genetics." They obviously have genetics that are capable of being healthy, because they are healthy. But, absent interventions to prevent them from consuming the Standard American Diet (SAD), they would likely struggle with weight. My wife and I both have extended families, like most Americans these days, with almost universal weight problems ranging from moderate to extreme. If my children resort to a Standard American Diet in adulthood, they might struggle with weight. I am hopeful, and there's evidence to suggest this is at least partly true, that if my children avoid weight problems in childhood, they are less likely to have weight problems as adults, even if their diets regress a little bit.

But that day, at a little Whataburger in Liberty, Texas, I realized, at least for the present moment, we had changed our family tree.

We do not live in a high-end zip code where a Dairy Queen is as rare as a cash-advance loan shark. They had this lack of experience with garbage food due to deliberate choices my wife and I had made over the past ten years or so. It had not always been this way.

My Moment of Realization

Have you ever had a moment where something you've been hiding from yourself suddenly became undeniable? With my weight, that happened for me in the spring of 2006. Someone snapped a photo:

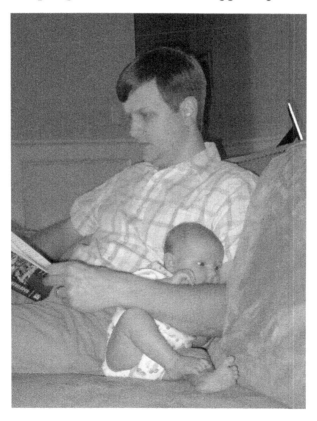

This photo was taken at an interesting moment in my life. I was about to turn twenty-seven, and we had just welcomed our second daughter, Olivia, to the family that spring. My business partners and I had the impeccable timing of getting distracted from our main business and trying our hand at real-estate development, buying a raw piece of land nearby in early 2006. Consistent with my personality, my first thought was to buy and read a textbook on the subject. So, here I am trying to multitask spending time with my infant and reading a book about my obsession of the moment. Here's another revealing picture from a few years earlier (and yes, most of the photos of me from this period are with babies):

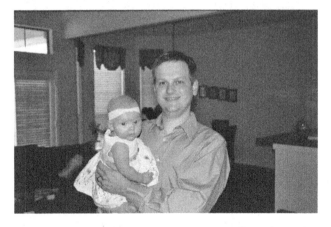

While I had struggled with weight off and on since childhood, this photo made my avoidance, my little evasions of my current state impossible to maintain.

Everyone who struggles with weight has these tricks. My favorite two were to suck in my gut when I looked in the mirror and to reassure myself that I wore "only" size 34, well maybe 36, pants. Interestingly, today my actual waist size is 34 inches, even though my pants say 31 inches. I was probably closer to 38 or 40 inches at this moment, young and healthy, but setting myself up for big problems later on.

I don't know what changed for me inside, but seeing this photo, I finally arrived at a determination to do whatever it took to improve my situation. A few years earlier I had quit my job to start a business, so I had complete control over my time and diet. I could afford to take time off in my day to exercise, and I could certainly afford whatever food I might need. I came to believe that I had absolutely no excuse for not changing, unless I wanted to admit that I was a weak person who could not control my animal appetites.

My weight had not always been this bad. I was chubby at times as a kid. I grew up at the height of the all-you-can-eat buffet chains–Ryan's, Golden Corral, Bonanza, Quincy's–and supersized fast-food meals. As I got taller in high school, I slimmed down to the point where I was not recognizably overweight, probably due to my involvement with marching band, which lasts almost all year long in my native state of Louisiana due to the Mardi Gras season. We marched in football games and in 14-mile-long parades in everything from heat to freezing sleet due to the schizophrenic Louisiana winters, in addition to after-school practice in 95 degree heat in the fall. Even though I didn't eat that well, my body was young enough that I slimmed up from the physical activity.

College was a different story. I had skipped a grade early in elementary school, so I went to college at Texas A&M, more than six hours from home, at barely seventeen years old. My required physical activity plunged while I became solely responsible for my nutrition with all-you-can-eat cafeterias as my primary food source. I made poor decisions and knew little to nothing about nutrition. This was the age of "low fat" dogma, so everyone thought soft drinks and cookies were A-okay as long as they were low fat. By the summer before my senior year, I had swelled to 190 pounds on my 5'10" frame. I was smack in the middle of the overweight range by BMI, halfway to obesity at barely twenty years old.

I managed to slim down to about 175 pounds by the following summer and fall, right before meeting and beginning to date my future wife. But, I still ate garbage on and off and my success was middling at best.

When I started my business, my partners and I stocked the office fridge with every possible variety of sugar drink, with a few diet drinks thrown in for balance. I thought myself reasonable for drinking only one Coca-Cola per day, the kind from Mexico with real sugar in the glass bottle that was supposed to be healthier. I kept growing after the birth of my first child, to the point where I got close to my college peak again, north of 180 pounds. Then this photo peeled away the lies I had been telling myself, and I finally became serious about losing the weight once and for all.

Over the next year, I was able to reduce my weight to under 160 pounds and my pant size to 31 inches, and have maintained this for over a decade. While my previous obesity probably means I will never have visible "abs"–I tried, and they still didn't show up even when I wasted myself to below 150 pounds–I was happy with the way I looked. For the first time I could remember, I was not self-conscious about taking off my shirt in public.

Here's a picture from recent years:

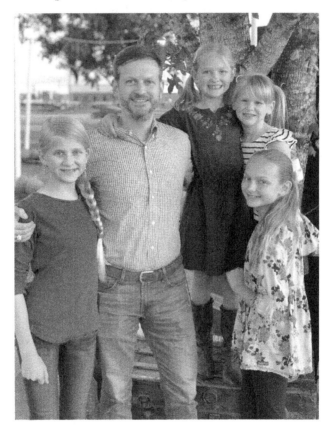

How did I do it? At the time I didn't think it was anything remarkable. At first, I cut myself to one-half a Coca-Cola per day, then switched to a cola with lower sugar, and finally dropped the habit altogether. However, my main breakthrough was stumbling across something that worked for me better than I could imagine: boring food.

I've always been a fan of efficiency and avoiding needless daily decisions which burn mental energy and willpower. I was too lazy to actually count calories, so instead I ate mostly the same things to make the counting easier. I standardized on the same breakfast every morning, either a protein shake or a high-fiber cereal with milk. I purchased limited-calorie frozen meals in the 400 to 500 calorie range, and rotated the same five to ten meals for my lunch every day. If you've ever had "diet" frozen meals, you know they're pretty boring tasting.

At night, I didn't allow myself seconds. I also didn't allow myself snacks at night. I made a rule that if I was hungry, I could eat, but I had to eat fruit: nothing else was on the menu. I limited dessert to about once a week, and cut down my portions of sweets to half typical size.

While my motivation for doing this was to avoid the prep, calculations, and hassle of counting every calorie, the boring part was more important than I appreciated at the time. It just worked, and I would only learn why later as I delved into the biochemistry and neuroscience of food and addiction.

Why We Overeat

The "low fat" dogma of the 1980s and '90s was so obviously wrong—it didn't work for most, and as Americans cut their fat intake, they got fatter—it's no wonder so many diet fads sprung up to fill the gap: Sugar Busters, Low Carb, Atkins, Zone, Whole Food, Keto, Gluten Free, Intermittent Fasting. Many of these worked better than the mainstream advice, at least for a time.

However, all of them had issues with adherence. We all have the friend who gets super pumped about low carb, loses ten or twenty pounds, and then puts all the weight back on in a year. The problem is that low carb is really hard to stick to for the long term.

Sugar Busters might have been the closest to the truth, while Zone allowed junk food of all kinds as long as macros were balanced. Gluten-free cut out the temptation of bread, but once the gluten-free "industry" started pumping out the same garbage food with potato and rice starch, many former gluten eaters ended up worse off than before. Atkins worked for many at first, but people gravitated to the least boring foods on the menu, like bacon, sausage, and artificially sweetened sodas, instead of the steak, chicken, and broccoli the good doctor originally intended.

Donald Trump once famously said, when the winner of one of his beauty pageants gained 30 pounds in the months following the competition, that "she likes to eat." This really is why we overeat: we like it too much. Trump himself could take his same advice these days–though his ego would never let him admit it, he's probably the second fattest President in American history.

Sometimes you have to tell it like it is. Americans are literally addicted to junk food. We like it, and we don't want to stop.

Why do alcoholics drink? They like getting drunk and feeling the buzz that melts away all of life's anxieties. They like getting drunk more than the consequences of being a drunk.

Why do heroin users shoot up? They like the overwhelming high that washes over them and all of their troubles like a wave of warm water. They like the feeling of being high more than life itself.

Why do people overeat? Junk food makes them feel good, and they prefer these feelings to the short-term and long-term negative consequences of obesity.

Why does junk food make us feel so good? An emerging area in biology is the study of supernormal stimuli. The theory is that our brain uses certain shortcuts to make decisions that are normally beneficial, but these decisions can be harmful in artificial, modern environments. Birds, for example, can be enticed to abandon their eggs if presented with a larger, more brightly colored egg. The bird's brain uses the shortcut of brightly-colored, largish, oblong objects to identify her eggs, and when presented with a similar stimulus that is artificially amplified, she prefers the stimulus to the real thing.

Human brains take similar shortcuts. When presented with tasty high-fat, high-carbohydrate foods, our survival instinct tells us we must eat as much as possible. Given the risk of famine for most of human history, this was a useful part of our design; if we could make ourselves overeat before food became scarce, we would be more likely to survive. Today, however, famine is mostly not a concern, absent entirely in the developed world and almost eliminated in the developing world. This design feature has become a liability.

Americans may have a double problem here. Because our country was so spread out, with a hotter climate and lower population density than Europe, we lost many of the healthier Old World food traditions. Few Americans of the 19th century could walk to town daily to purchase fresh baguettes, fresh meat, fresh dairy, etc. It was either made on the farm or available as a processed food. Americans invented fake chocolate and fake cheese, for example, because of the difficulty of storing and transporting fresh food to distant markets. As a result, many food traditions in the United States are intimately tied to junk food. We are emotionally tied to the stuff in ways other cultures are not.

The solution is not easy, but it's simple. We simply have to eat less food that we really like, and more food we are indifferent about. Like a drug user, I had to hit rock bottom, seeing that photo, to desire to change my ways more than continuing them. But unlike a drug user, I can't simply quit eating. Food is strange in that it is both a necessary thing for life and also an abusable pleasure. The inability to go "cold turkey" makes quitting food abuse harder in some ways, but easier in others. We can change the desirability of the food we eat, and thereby extinguish the addictive part of our relationship with it.

This required I come to terms with a hard truth about myself: food was way too important to me. In religious terms, it became an idol, more important to me than building up the temple of my body. To kill food's power over me, I had to kill my desire for it, which meant strictly limiting desirable foods.

Man has always wanted to denigrate the role of the body and see himself as a spirit independent of it. We see this in everything from the functional Gnosticism of many churches that elevates the spirit over the physical to the secular hope of immortality imagined by Silicon Valley moguls who want to "upload" their brains to the data cloud. In Christian theology, we are told that human beings will have bodies, forever. Taking care of the body we have now is a preparation for eternity.

Just like drug abuse, food abuse is partially a spiritual problem. We get confused because the observable manifestations are more physical, but the root spiritual cause is the same: a love of temporary pleasure over our duties to ourselves, God, and our fellow man.

However, it is not solely a spiritual problem. The spiritual part is acknowledging the problem and a determination to fight it and do whatever it takes to defeat it, assuming such a defeat is possible. But, like drug addiction, it manifests physically as well, and once begun as a habit, it is harder to break once started than to avoid beforehand. This is why I'm so passionate about childhood obesity: like cigarettes, it's so much harder to quit than to never start.

Any one of us, if we had some serious accident or health problem where it became necessary, will become physiologically addicted to narcotic pain medicine within days or weeks. This physical process is not a spiritual failing any more than the biochemical reaction to any other medication. The problem is that so many of our foods are more addictive than nutritious, similar to narcotics. To apply our spiritual determination to break or avoid food abuse, we must understand these physical causes.

The Biochemistry of Food Addiction

I used to want to impress people with my vocabulary. As I've gotten older, I've become more skeptical of people who use big words needlessly. I now believe that if a person can't explain something in simple language, say at the level that a fourth grader could at least partially understand, he or she doesn't really understand it themselves. Part of my purpose in writing this is to make sure I know what I'm talking about and can organize all of my thoughts coherently, and I've challenged myself to do that in the simplest possible language. Too often complicated words hide vague ideas that don't mean anything.

One of my hobbies is reading science books, and I find nutritional science particularly fascinating. I've probably read all of the major popular science books on the subject published in the last ten years, including books advocating low carb, fasting, avoiding wheat, and counting calories. I think they're all correct in a sense, and I believe there is an overarching theory that explains how all of them get something right.

Unfortunately, the world of nutrition advice is something like a religion for a lot of people now. With a problematic mainstream consensus, people have separated into various camps, each with its own guru advocating a plausible solution. There's Gary Taubes and the low-carb, neo-Atkins camp. There's of course the old low-fat, high-fiber people, now also laced with a touch of veganism and environmental alarmism about meat.

If all of the popular diets get something right and work for many people while contradicting each other, what common factors could possibly explain why? The credit for that goes to Stephen Guyenet, a nutrition researcher and author of *The Hungry Brain*. I highly recommend the book if you want to go deeper, though it is heavy on science and light on application, for a specific reason I will explain later.

Guyenet highlights two experiments in his book that both challenge calorie-counting, eat-less-exercise-more mainstream advice, and low-carb/paleo dogma.

The first was a nutrition study where people were held in a hospital and served, for all of their meals, a nutritionally complete, bland, slightly sweet "goop." The subjects could eat as much of the goop as they wanted, at any time. This goop was not particularly healthy, having a good many high glycemic carbohydrates, a moderate amount of protein and fat, and some sugar. It was, however, very bland and of no recognizable flavor.

Link: https://tinyurl.com/goopstudy

The researchers recruited both non-overweight and overweight people for the study. The results? The healthy-weight people ate enough goop to maintain their weight, neither gaining nor losing. The overweight people, surprisingly, would only eat about 300 to 400 calories of the goop a day, feeling full after ingesting a minimal amount, and began to lose weight. Since almost every other study of allowing people to eat whatever they want reveals that overweight people eat more than skinny people–the folk wisdom of "metabolism" being the reason why people get fat doesn't account for much of the difference–this result was a bit of a mystery.

The second experiment involved rats, or rather involved scientific researchers trying to deliberately fatten rats to enable further experiments. It turns out it's extremely hard to make rats overeat, at least by standard methods. They tried adding more fat, carbohydrates, or sugar to their chow, with limited results. What actually worked to make rats fat? One of the researchers decided to start feeding some of the rats human junk food from the grocery store, such as candy, bread, mass market cheese, and cheap deli meats. Once given unlimited access to this stuff, the rats fattened up quickly.

Link: https://tinyurl.com/ratsjunkfood

If the low-carb zealots are right, what could possibly account for these results? The goop served to people in the first experiment was high carb, just not very tasty. And rats only succumbed to the temptation to stuff themselves when offered human food and did not get fat on high-carb rat chow. Clearly if carbs were the cause, both groups would have gained weight. The low-carb idea is not completely wrong, and I'll try to explain why I think it's half right later. But clearly these two experiments show there's yet another factor.

In a blow to "paleo" orthodoxy, Guyenet documents how groups of human hunter-gatherers live on an all kinds of macronutrient combinations, and none of them get fat on their natural foods. Yes, some tribes eat almost nothing but coconut and fish, but another equally non-overweight tribe in Africa regularly gets 70 to 80 percent of their calories from wild honey, which is almost pure sugar! Others live on starchy root vegetables, with meat only as an occasional supplement. Though varied across people groups, indigenous diets are internally universally boring (more on this later), usually comprising a few staples for the vast majority of calories.

Interestingly, very few hunter-gatherers eat many vegetables, as the return on energy investment of gathering and cooking the food isn't worth their time. You can't support our big brain's energy needs on a lettuce diet. It seems that human beings are omnivores of all naturally-occurring calorie-dense foods, because no matter what natural diet hunter-gatherers consume, they don't get fat. The minute, however, they get access to the infinite tasty varieties of Western junk food, they start putting on weight. It's about more than carbs.

Guyenet takes the reader on a tour of biochemistry, moving up the chain of causation from insulin in the body to leptin in the brain. Leptin was discovered in the 1990s as the hormone that serves as a master control for hunger–as a person of normal weight eats, leptin increases, and then they feel full and stop eating. Perhaps overweight people had a leptin deficiency. It was thought that if we could just give overweight people more leptin, perhaps as a medicine, they would stop being as hungry and naturally lose weight.

Things in the body are rarely that simple. Looking into it further, researchers found that overweight people actually had *higher* levels of leptin than normal people. Leptin worked normally in people of healthy weight, rising when they ate and killing off hunger quickly. But in overweight people, it didn't work the same way. Leptin levels had to get a lot higher in the overweight group before the hunger subsided. Just as pre-diabetics have extremely high levels of insulin, but their cells stop responding to it, overweight people, long before they become diabetic, become **resistant** to the effects of leptin. They ate more and were hungrier doing so, and they only got full after eating a lot more food to get leptin levels high enough for their brain to respond.

This concept of "resistance" is key to understanding this research. A good analogy is that of hearing damage. When people get exposed to really loud levels of noise, their auditory nerve cells become overstimulated and eventually stop responding as much to sound. If it goes on long enough, loud volumes start to sound normal, and hearing becomes very difficult at normal or quiet levels. Hearing aids only put a band-aid on the problem by amplifying ambient sound.

It appears that really tasty human foods are so enjoyable that the body starts to ignore the leptin signal to stop eating. This makes sense, as we've all had the experience of having that "second stomach" for dessert or a savory, salty snack even though we have no remaining desire to eat healthy food. But, as people keep eating these tasty foods, leptin levels keep going up. If they stay high enough for long enough, the brain gets trained to partially ignore the leptin signal. Once it does that, the body is only satisfied with higher food intake before it will stop being hungry, which leads to weight gain, except in those who have the exceptional self-control to tolerate constant hunger.

The good news is that it appears the body can regain leptin sensitivity. The "goop" experiment shows what happens when the reward of food is taken away and nutrition is provided in an extremely boring, monotonous form. Healthy-weight people keep eating normally, because their primary relationship with food is that of biological necessity. They eat when hungry, leptin goes up, and they stop eating. When leptin drops again, they eat, even eating unappealing food if necessary, to maintain weight.

I have made an interesting observation of friends of mine who have been slim all their life. Often, when going out to eat, they will order more than I expect, perhaps an appetizer, a big entrée and a dessert. I can see why the typical overweight person might think life unfair, and assume the difference must be something like genetics or metabolism. But observe closely, and you'll see that these naturally slim people pick at their food. They eat a bit of the appetizer, leaving most of it behind. They leave much of the entrée, and they maybe eat half the dessert. Maybe they take the leftovers home, but sometimes they just leave them on the table. They're full, and they stop eating. Slim people are strangely indifferent to food.

The overweight, however, have a primary relationship with food that is based on pleasure, not biological need. Take the pleasure away but keep the nutrition, and suddenly the brain starts paying more attention to the elevated leptin levels. Deprived of pleasure in food, the overweight person eats **less** than the healthy-weight person. Why? Because absent that addictive pleasure, the overweight person's body starts to listen to the leptin signal again–remember the overweight have **higher** leptin levels–resulting in a massive drop in food intake, as if the body has finally "woken up" to the fact that there are extra fat stores it would prefer to "eat" instead of the unappealing, bland food choices. With no pleasure available, only nutrition, the body chooses to eat less and start moving towards a healthy weight.

This is the key to the mystery of why all diets work, at least somewhat. Whether low-fat or low-carb, no popular guru is promoting a junk food diet. Every single diet regime involves getting rid of junk food, at least in theory, and practiced this way, it seems to matter very little whether what is eaten is bland oatmeal or scrambled eggs. Neither food is that rewarding compared to junk food.

There's a saying in business that once a metric becomes a target, it's no longer a useful metric. This creates a situation where the smart manager will have certain favorite numbers to monitor to see what's going on in a business, but will not set these numbers as goals for the organization. The metric can indicate possible opportunities for further investigation, but once you incentivize people to hit a certain metric as a target, they change their behavior in strange ways to hit a number without changing or improving the harder-to-measure behaviors that went into the metric originally.

The same thing happens to every diet program that gets popular enough. Atkins and low-carb worked wonders for many people, until food manufacturers caught up with the trend and started making low-carb junk food—candy bars, cookies, almond chips, you name it. Very few low-carb people are eating chicken breast, sirloin steak, and broccoli. Many are eating low-carb junk food, or hyper-palatable, easy-to-prepare processed meats like bacon or sausage. Weight loss stalls once the body finds a substitute addiction that checks the low-carb box.

I said earlier that low carb was half right. Eating too many calories for too long results in insulin resistance. Insulin is the body's master hormone for regulating blood sugar. Too much of it and our body drains the blood of its glucose, shunting it into fat cells, leaving the body fatter and hungrier at the same time. This adds to the hunger of the pre-existing leptin resistance. It could be that short-term leptin resistance from eating what Guyenet calls "hyper-palatable" food eventually leads to insulin resistance. Once someone has insulin resistance, that becomes another problem to fix. And no doubt, ketogenic and other low-carb diets are the best treatment for insulin resistance, often leading to a complete reversal of diabetes.

The low-carb folks are partially right for one other very strong reason. Guyenet identifies two types of particularly hyper-palatable foods: flavored, liquid sugar (i.e. sodas) and high-fat, high-carb foods, particularly those combining sugar and fat. These two combinations seem to "hack" our brains' ability to limit itself to reasonable amounts of food.

By strictly limiting carbohydrates, at a first pass the low-carb regime eliminates the primary source of food that makes us overeat, not because they're carbs per-se, but because they taste better to us than low-carb options. It turns out that it's really hard to get fat on fat and protein alone, because the food is not nearly as appealing in the same quantities as those containing combinations of sugar, carbohydrates, and fat.

How can we apply Guyenet's findings? His book is really short on practical recommendations, mostly because I think he realizes no one wants his solutions. Or maybe because he's so smart it seems obvious to him. He's an intelligent guy, interested in the science, and probably finds the application part a bit boring. I'm here to provide the practical solution based on Guyenet's scientific model.

The solution is what I call The Boring Diet.

The Boring Diet

My successful long-term weight loss required a complete overhaul of how and when I ate. My relationship with food had to move from a place where pleasure and experience were central to a place where I ate in response to my true biological needs.

Normally, weight loss involves a lot of hunger. Humans are not good at resisting hunger in the long run. But the "goop" experiment showed that weight loss was possible without hunger, as long as the food is boring enough. How does this get applied to real life?

I'll start off with the negative part of the diet, the stuff we cannot have in our immediate environment while maintaining or transitioning to a healthy weight, along with a simple system for hunger management. Mostly, this is a strategy for dealing with snacking, which is where most weight gain takes place.

Luckily, the human hunger system is pretty primitive. It's not very smart, and it can be easily defeated by the thinking part of the brain. One breakthrough method of addiction treatment enabling people to immediately pursue abstinence without resorting to the melodrama of the XYZ

"Anonymous" movements is something called Addictive Voice Recognition Therapy (AVRT).

Related to cognitive behavioral therapy, AVRT helps people depersonalize their addictive drives. The approach advises people to call their addictive drives a "beast," using the pronoun "it" to refer to it internally. Instead of saying "I'm hungry for some ice cream," clients are taught to say "It is hungry for ice cream."

It is the precise opposite of the AA approach, which encourages people to identify their core selves with their addiction. AVRT says, no, you are so much more as a human being than your addiction. In fact, the entire process of addiction is simply a cognitive-behavioral error, something false that is learned, and can be unlearned. The false belief is that the destructive addictive drive represents something profound about one's true self, and that to leave the addiction would be to give up a part of one's identity. This is not the case. The addictive drives are from the dumb animal part of our brains and can be dealt with on that basis.

What I'm saying is that your appetite has more in common with a dog's appetite than it does with the creative and executive functions of your mind. It is persuasive, but only because it pretends to be part of you, when it is, in fact, not a central part of the personality.

To explore this in more detail, see the framework at the AVRT website:

Link: https://tinyurl.com/feastbeast

We can utilize the appetite's lack of intelligence to structure our lives to minimize hunger while losing or maintaining weight. Let me get to the point: this animal drive is much more concerned with immediate pleasure that anything else. It wants junk food, and it wants it now. Deprive it of junk food and make tasty food higher effort, and it will quiet down, just like it did for those eating the "goop."

Excessive hunger for those already overweight is nothing more than the animal response to the availability of junk food in the everyday environment. Eliminate the junk food–get it out of the house, away from your desk, and in the trash– and we're halfway to eliminating the hunger normally required to lose weight.

How do I define junk food? Simple: it's any food you like a whole lot that can be eaten with minimal effort. Mostly, that's processed, packaged food. You must ruthlessly go through your home and work environments and eliminate all of these kinds of foods.

Foods to Definitely Eliminate from Your Environment

- Candy, chips, cookies. They must go to the trash and never return to your environment.

- Soda. Eliminating all sweetened beverages is perhaps your highest leverage opportunity. They only stimulate pleasure while doing little to shut off the drive to eat. This includes artificially sweetened drinks as well. No one really knows why, but they're even worse than sugary drinks, according to numerous studies. One theory is that the body knows it's being tricked, and so seeks more sugar later. Another theory is that these chemicals are more toxic than we think, and biological systems are more complex than we think, so they could be hurting us without us understanding why quite yet. Remember how for many years we were told that trans fats in margarine and Crisco were better for us than animal fat, yet later we discovered a mechanism by which trans fats directly cause heart disease? They're certainly not necessary, and even if it turns out they're safe, they're risky based on the current science. Plus, they taste good, and part of The Boring Diet is to eat less food that stimulates hunger. Don't drink sugar or artificial sugar substitutes.

- Breads. Some of the anti-wheat people speculate that wheat contains "opioid peptides" that make bread especially addictive. The idea is that the reason we like bread is because it makes us high, like a drug. I don't know enough to say if this is true or not, but I do know that wheat breads are a major temptation. When I was fat and in the absence of real junk food, a slice of bread or two would do in a pinch. And when bread is offered at the table, I'm more tempted to have seconds than with other starches like rice. Rice and potatoes are mostly whole foods, with the cell walls of the plant largely still intact. This may limit the rate at which they produce pleasure in the gut from spiking the blood sugar. Wheat flour, on the other hand, is a powdered starch, which is absorbed almost immediately. It's like the difference between wine and hard liquor.

- Juice. Juice is sugar and flavor removed from the fiber of a fruit. Sugar itself is basically dried sugar cane juice. Eliminate all juice.

- Highly sweetened dairy products. Whether it's yogurt or coffee drinks, if you have bottles of this stuff on-hand ready to consume, you will eat it. Get rid of it. It's all gotta go, even stuff with sophistication halos like Starbucks Frappuccinos.

- Granola bars, "snack bars," and the like. Again, if it's convenient and you like it, it must go.

- Ice cream and all ready-to-eat desserts. You know this has to go; it's too tempting for a late night binge.

- Cereals and other ready-to-eat breakfast carbs. Cereal consists of highly-processed grains spiked with sugar. This "part of a healthy breakfast" is just another excuse to eat dessert, and most have negligible protein, critical to controlling hunger early in the day. They're also way too easy to grab for a tasty snack. Put them all in the trash.

Foods to Possibly Eliminate

- Salted nuts. From talking to people who have tried or encouraged others to do low-carb diets, nuts seem like a common source of failing. When you've eliminated chips, cookies, etc, sometimes the animal appetite will latch onto nuts as its next fix. While nuts in moderation are very healthy, salted, or even worse, honey roasted type nuts, can be extremely hard to resist. If you are eating more than one serving a day, get rid of them or replace with unsalted nuts, which are not nearly the same temptation.

- Dried fruit. While I recommend whole fruit as one of The Boring Diet boring snacking options, dried fruit may present some issues. Dates and raisins, stripped of their natural water, are extremely high sugar per serving, even if technically there's no sugar added. Dried cranberries are really candied cranberries, since sugar must be added to the tart fruit to make them tolerably sweet. If these are a temptation, remove them.

- Sausage and bacon. This is heresy among the low-carb crowd, but these foods are very tasty, heavily processed, and high in calories. If you like them too much, they can wreck the goal of weight loss on a lower carb diet.

- Healthy "junk food." If you have a problem overeating protein bars, they have to go. If you like semi-healthy bars like KIND bars or RXBARs too much, they have to go. If granola or even "grain free" granola is a snacking problem, it needs to go. We want to completely eliminate all super tasty convenience eating.

This seems pretty extreme, I know. But these are all foods our ancestors would never have eaten. Convenient, pre-packaged, shelf-stable, tasty food simply didn't exist. Yet this extremity is very necessary, as we get to the central premise of this book:

Hunger is relative.

The animal inside of me wants me to think that hunger represents a non-negotiable, absolute biological need that I must address or die. More realistically, though, it's a symptom of the lust my appetite has for an immediate hit of tasty junk food. When you remove the junk from your environment, taking away its opportunity for a quick payoff, you'll find you're a lot less hungry.

Remember the goop experiment. Absent tasty food with a pleasurable payoff, the biological need for food is very limited for the overweight person. The body knows at some level it has too much excess fat, but it doesn't want to give up any of it as long as tasty junk food is available. If the "tomorrow" never comes, it never gives up the fat.

I just cannot emphasize enough how important, absolutely critical, it is to eliminate this stuff from the home and work environment. **Hunger is relative.** You're hungry because you eat these foods and they taste too good. You eat them despite your best intentions because they are in your immediate environment.

This is super simple but not easy. So far, we've covered half the strategy: eliminate convenient, tasty food. Hunger naturally goes down. But it's not gone. What do we do with the hunger that still torments us, negotiates with us, tempts us to drive to the store and replenish our inventory of addictive foods?

Surprise: we feed the hunger, just not with what it wants. There's a famous cartoon where Donald Duck's nephews, Huey, Dewey, and Louie, are caught smoking cigarettes. Their punishment: Uncle Scrooge makes them smoke the whole pack at once, until they are so sick of cigarettes they want to vomit. Take the novelty and turn it into monotony.

We often get the idea that changing one's weight is really hard. Yet, massive weight gain and loss happens all the time in Hollywood. Actress Charlize Theron, 5'10", gained 50 pounds for her role in the movie *Tully*. She also took it back off again when the filming was over and went back to her normal, healthy weight. In an interview on *Ellen* she revealed how she gained the weight:

> "I ate a lot of everything, but my drug of choice is potato chips. I ate them everywhere. I had a bag in my car, a bag in the bathroom, a bag in the kitchen, a bag on the counter, a

bag in my trailer. Everywhere I went there was just a bag."

She did the opposite of The Boring Diet. She ate a tasty food and made it super convenient to consume. This also implies that potato chips are not a normal part of her food environment, and that she is not simply genetically gifted with an ability to eat whatever she wants and not gain weight.

Actor Joaquin Phoenix similarly lost 52 pounds for his role in 2019's *Joker*, starving himself to nearly anorexic levels of body fat for the role.

It turns out that people can lose and gain weight, and lose it again, pretty easily when their income depends on it. For an actor, actress, or model, weighing the right amount for the role is simply part of the job. Part of the problem is that people see losing weight as optional. When it's not optional, when millions of dollars and one's livelihood is on the line, it turns out that people can gain and lose pretty easily.

We need to get into the mental space of treating eating like a job, instead of recreation. All functional adults learn the difference between work and recreation. I learned it early shortly after my fifteenth birthday, just after getting my license. My Dad had arranged with a high school buddy of his who managed the local supermarket for me to begin a job bagging groceries, gathering carts, and doing general cleanup. I wasn't asked whether I wanted this job. I was expected to show up.

I learned quickly to like, but not love, my work. While it wasn't exactly recreation, the sense of rhythm of the work day, and the busyness of the store, made time pass quickly. And after a shift, there was the sense of accomplishment in having done something tangible and earned a paycheck.

Our relationship with food needs to be more like our mentality at work than the mentality we have when we recreate. It's a job to feed our bodies appropriately to achieve a long-term goal. The essence of work is to put off immediate gratification to serve someone else. The essence of a healthy diet is to put off gratification to serve your future self. What difference should it make whether you're getting paid to do it? Sure, Hollywood professionals have their paychecks on the line, but isn't your health more important to you than money is to them?

These professionals have the same biological systems as you or me. Reading about their techniques, they simply have two things most people don't: a necessity to get it done because a paycheck depends on it, and some effective techniques for doing so. From reading about their techniques, one stands out in particular: the eating of bland, low-calorie food to fight hunger. Apples, carrot sticks, turkey slices, all of these seem to figure prominently in the snacking diets of those who must stay in shape for a living.

The second part of The Boring Diet strategy is to pick a monotonous, boring, bland, low-calorie food to give the animal inside when it demands to be fed. For me, what seemed to work was to only allow myself to snack on whole fruit. I was a night snacker. After an evening meal, I felt entitled to some late-night chips and salsa, or a bowl of "light" ice cream, or perhaps some peanut butter and crackers. Besides Mexican Cokes during the workday, these 400 to 500 calorie "bonus meals" at night were my downfall. I almost always wanted them regardless of my true level of hunger because it felt good to eat them. Fruit, however, for me, was boring.

So when my appetite told me it wanted some peanut butter and crackers, I responded internally like this: "I understand you are hungry and it is never my intention to starve you, my beloved body, nor to harm you with foods that will hurt us in the long-term. So, if as you claim, you are desperately hungry, I will feed you some apple slices." Amazingly, after an apple or two, more often just one, the hunger went away.

This is similar to a strategy that will be familiar to many parents. Kids often complain about being hungry outside of mealtimes because kids have even less self-control than adults. Smart parents will say something like, "You may have a banana." What the kid really wants is some kind of junk food, but more times than not, when offered the banana, the kid turns it down. And if they want the banana, great, they were legitimately hungry and were given legitimately healthy food. It's truly a win-win offer.

We are playing the same psychological trick on our primitive, child-like hunger instinct. We have removed all of the immediate temptations that cause it to throw temper tantrums, and when it still whines it is hungry, we provide it with sustenance. Boring, healthy sustenance. Like apples. Or bananas. Or deli turkey breast slices. And if you're really aggressive, carrots, which have a negligible number of calories after the energy spent digesting them. Basically, the appetite gets fed, but it doesn't get rewarded. The conditioning of food addiction is being broken. I had to subdue my flesh which wanted to eat crap for short-term pleasure hits that would eventually kill me. You must do the same.

These go-to, unexciting snacks for killing hunger can be remembered by the acronym BCAT: if hungry, you may have a banana, carrots, apple slices, or turkey. These are all dirt cheap at the grocery store and are low calorie and nutritious. BCAT all day long and you'll never go hungry. You might get bored, but you won't be hungry. It's called The Boring Diet for a reason.

Why does this method work? What's going on in the brain?

One of the most effective techniques for treating alcoholism is the Sinclair Method. Developed by Dr. David Sinclair, and tested for effectiveness in Finland, the Sinclair Method involves encouraging alcoholics to drink when they would like, but with one simple rule. An hour before they drink anything, they must take a dose of a drug called Naltrexone.

Naltrexone is an opioid blocker. Opioids exist naturally in our body and make us feel good after exercise, or after a really rich dessert. Opioids can be taken artificially by taking opioid drugs, some of the most addictive known to man, but they're also stimulated by drinking alcohol. Alcohol feels good because the "buzz" is our body's own opiates being stimulated by the presence of ethanol.

With naltrexone, even though alcohol has all of its normal negative side effects–drowsiness, poor motor control, impaired thinking–it does not produce a "buzz." In Sinclair's view, all addiction is a function of a learning process. We drink too much, or eat too much, because we learn to do so. When the pleasure of alcohol is removed, the learned behavior–drinking alcohol–is "extinguished," in psychological terms. Just as a fire is extinguished without oxygen or fuel, learned addictions are extinguished when the payoff of pleasure is separated from the addictive behavior.

Strangely, Sinclair's method works a lot better when alcoholics take naltrexone **only** before drinking instead of daily. We actually don't want the opioid receptors blocked all the time, just when the addictive behavior might occur. And when deprived of the addictive pleasure, the opiate receptors become more sensitive to other stimuli. When not drinking, this gives new, non-destructive behaviors a chance to replace the addictive behavior. This new learning replaces the old, harmful learning, and the former alcoholic can be conditioned to be almost indifferent to his former vice.

When it comes to food, we have to eat so often that it isn't practical to take a drug like naltrexone to decondition our pleasure response to junk food. By replacing junk foods, particularly snacks, with bland, healthy food, something similar is accomplished. The learned behavior–eating– becomes ever more disconnected from the former pleasures of super tasty food.

What You Should Eat

I covered the "what not to eat" part first because it is the most critical component of this system. When it comes to what you should eat, the main thing is to eat highly nutritious, high-protein meals that are calorie controlled.

I wrote about the merits of the low-carb diet earlier in this book, and I think a modified version of this, "lower processed carb" for lack of a better word, is best, particularly if you want weight loss that keeps working past the early momentum where nearly any approach works. We're not doing this because carbs are nutritionally "evil" in the body, but because our brains tend to overvalue carbohydrates, particularly when accompanied with sugar and/or fat. Here's how it's done:

- Don't eat any of the junk categories listed previously. All of them are ripe for abuse.

- Eat generally lower carbohydrate meals. Eat lots of lean meat. Prefer non-starchy vegetables over starchy vegetables.

- Eat eggs for breakfast, ideally two or three. Follow Tim Ferriss' advice to eat 30 grams of protein within thirty minutes of waking up, and do it with minimal calories. Three eggs and a low-fat Greek yogurt gets it done.

- Once or twice a day, it is acceptable to have rice or some sort of baked or roasted potato. Neither starch, as relatively unprocessed foods, are strongly associated with obesity.

- Avoid all fried foods. Battered fried food is one of those carb/fat pleasure bombs our brain really likes too much. Also, most of us are not frying at home with high smoke point fats like beef tallow or coconut oil. Because frying is so messy (and expensive, if the grease is not reused), most fried foods are eaten out, not in the home. Restaurants use commodity-grade soybean oil and they rarely change it out. These kinds of seed-based, polyunsaturated frying oils are extremely unstable chemically and break down into all kinds of nasty substances. Old, nasty soybean oil will cause massive inflammation in your body, besides the empty extra calories.

- Include beans in your diet. This again comes from Tim Ferriss with his "slow carb" diet. Guyenet, the nutrition science researcher, is a big fan of the Instant Pot for easily and quickly making batches of beans and other bland foods. Beans, like baked and roasted potatoes, appear to lower hunger despite having significant carbohydrates.

- To borrow from Ferriss again, he recommends, and I strongly endorse, eating similar foods for breakfast and lunch. Eat the same breakfast every day, and eat a boring lunch. Low-calorie high-protein frozen meals make this possible. You don't have to eat the same exact item every day, but the general taste of these products is bland enough that they satisfy hunger without stimulating it. Plus, portion and calorie control is built in and "done for you."

- One area where I disagree with Ferriss is his advocacy for "cheat days." These may work for active men with high muscle mass like Ferriss, but many will struggle with this tactic. It stimulates the appetite for the foods that cause hunger. You don't need a cheat day because real life will ensure you don't always stick to a boring diet perfectly. Alcoholics and drug addicts need as much abstinence as they can muster, not cheat days. The same goes for food addictions.

All weight loss necessarily involves eating fewer calories than you burn. The goal is to eat fewer calories with less hunger so the losses are sustainable. The reason to restrict certain foods is because they make us hungrier while adding substantially to the day's calories. We must achieve a sustainable calorie deficit.

The dieter also must not cut protein intake, as studies have shown that cutting calories in general will reduce muscle mass substantially, making weight maintenance more difficult, but extra protein will help spare muscle tissue. We need at least 0.5 grams per pound of body weight.

When all the variables are combined together–the need for a real calorie deficit, avoiding hunger-stimulating foods, and adequate protein intake–there are only a few paths to success. It mostly means eating protein-rich, lean or moderately lean foods, and a few unprocessed carbohydrates.

The Heart of the Boring Diet

The heart of The Boring Diet is it being boring. We pick foods that don't stimulate hunger very much, and we eat the same ones every day, as much as possible.

Even if we eliminate junk food, we can still stimulate our hunger with too much variety of healthy foods. Americans 100 years ago did not have anywhere near the variety of foods available to them as we do today in our local supermarkets. A lot of our ancestors ate very monotonous diets, especially when most areas had at most one or two staple crops. Some have theorized that the reason we are tempted by variety is that variety was typically only available at harvest time. This served as a signal for us to fatten up before winter, when variety would become scarce. Except today, "winter"–in terms of food supply and variety–never comes.

To lose fat without significant hunger, we must both eliminate foods that are inherently hunger producing **and** reduce variety of foods. We are laying a siege on the addictive animal inside to unlearn the addictive behavior until it no longer has a hold on us.

The Boring Diet means eating mostly the same food every day until the evening meal. The menus below are an optimized suggestion, but the monotony of The Boring Diet is its primary strength. If you're still making decisions for multiple meals a day about what you're eating, you're not following The Boring Diet.

Suggested Menus

I'll take a couple of examples and build from there. As a rule of thumb, a good weight loss diet is about 10 calories per pound of body weight, and at least 0.5 grams of protein per pound of body weight.

Fair or not, men can eat more than women and still lose weight, so I will specify the female diet and then add modifications for men.

Disclaimer: Women who are athletes, men who are athletes, or women who are breastfeeding tend to require a higher-calorie intake than people who are sedentary. This book is a narrative of strategies that worked for the author. Always consult a medical professional before beginning any diet or exercise program.

Standard Menu

Target: 1500 calories, 75 grams protein for a 150 pound woman

Let's start with breakfast, the easiest meal of the day to make monotonous and boring. My recommendation:

Breakfast: Three eggs, 225 calories, 21 grams of protein;YQ, Oikos Triple Zero, or Chobani Lower Sugar Greek Yogurt, 130 calories, 15 grams of protein

For breakfast, our subject has eaten only 355 calories and 36 grams of protein. This will be key to combating hunger for the rest of the day.

Lunch: For lunch, let's add a Healthy Choice "Simply Steamer" meal or something similar. This is about 230 calories, with 19 grams of protein.

Next, at 4:00 p.m., we add in a secret weapon. Recall earlier the key role protein plays in preventing the loss of muscle mass. One popular theory about why we overeat is that the body is just trying to get enough protein to support daily body repair processes, and it eats until it gets what it needs. If we eat low-protein foods, we have to eat more calories to get the necessary protein. This theory is probably partially true, as studies have shown that protein is both the least fattening and most filling. Protein is 4 calories per gram, just like carbohydrates, but the body has to burn more calories to convert it into fat storage. Protein intake alone has been shown to reduce hunger.

4:00 p.m. Shake: So at 4:00 p.m. every day, we are going to add in a whey protein shake. This accomplishes a few things. First, protein shakes don't taste that great, so it's akin to eating the "goop" that helps break the connection between sustenance and pleasure. While you will probably not enjoy the shake all that much while eating it, my experience has been that it does make me feel, more than any other food, a sense of satisfied, holistic fullness. This is because whey is the most complete- and easily-absorbed protein we can eat.

Second, we add more protein to the diet, which itself is necessary for healthy, sustainable fat loss. Third, we further standardize the diet and make predictable and "boring" most of the calories for the day. Fourth, we strategically kill hunger (and the pleasure of relieving that hunger with tasty food) before the evening meal, the only meal on the diet where decisions must be made about what and how much to eat. In a sense, whey protein serves as the dieter's naltrexone, killing hunger (and the pleasure of relieving it, like scratching an itch) before the more pleasurable evening meal.

For reference purposes, I'll use Tera's Whey Vanilla Protein Powder, made according to the label with water and/or ice. It is 110 calories, 21 grams of protein. This is extremely easy to do at work or on-the-go with a standard protein shaker.

Let's add up where we are so far:

Breakfast: 355 calories, 36 grams protein

Lunch: 230 calories, 19 grams protein

4:00 p.m. Shake: 110 calories, 21 grams protein

Low Calorie Snacks: BCAT—bananas, carrots, apples, turkey as needed to kill hunger

Total Before Evening Meal (not counting BCAT snacks): 695 calories, 76 grams protein

These are incredible statistics to be entering the "danger zone" of the evening meal. If the dieter will exercise basic self-control (avoiding forbidden foods and eating from the allowed foods list), it would be hard not to lose weight on such a diet. With a budget of 700 to 800 calories for the evening meal, one can go to bed satisfied.

Evening Meal: Let's say the evening meal is 700 calories and contains 25 grams of protein. Now we finish the day at 1395 calories and 101 grams of protein. That leaves about 100 calories for snacks, but don't worry about that. You will have a hard time eating enough whole apples and turkey breast to make a measurable impact. Even if you exceed the specified caloric limits, because of the types of food eaten, weight loss will still likely result, perhaps for reasons we don't quite understand. Perhaps eliminating leptin resistance itself accelerates fat loss, or stimulates physical activity due to excess energy. The calorie limits also have some flex, and will work even with some overage.

The evening meal is a definite temptation. The animal inside will be looking for this area of discretion to undo the day's progress. You must make yourself eat a reasonable portion of food. If you fill up a standard plate with standard servings with items not on the forbidden food list, it should be hard to exceed 700 calories.

What is a standard serving? For fatty meat, a deck of cards. For lean meat, two decks of cards. For starches, it's about half the size of a baseball. For non-starchy vegetables, a baseball. Though for the latter—broccoli, green beans, etc.—you could have more since the calorie density is so low. The main thing to limit is the fatty meat and starches to reasonable portions. This discretion, however, is hard. If you struggle with limiting the evening meal to a protein-rich 700-800 calories, it may be helpful to utilize a food tracking tool like MyFitnessPal. Though The Boring Diet is designed to work without calorie counting, or more precisely the counting in done in advance with pre-planned food for most of the day, it can be helpful to count calories for a while to recalibrate your own expectations of what a reasonable evening meal should look like.

Remember you do not have to be hungry. Eat a reasonable meal within the calorie limit, then offer yourself something from the BCAT menu as needed to fill the gap.

Also remember that The Boring Diet has some give and take built-in where it should work even with imperfect adherence at night. Because so much of the rest of the day is perfectly controlled, pre-ordained food that stays the same, 75 percent of the hard work is already done by the time you get to the evening meal. And if you slip, there's no decisions to make until the following evening. Especially early in the process, you can do this imperfectly and still lose a ton of weight if you follow a fixed, boring diet during the day.

Scaling the Diet Up or Down

For men, the portions are going to have to scale up by about one-third. So for a 200 pound man, we would modify as follows to add even more protein and get to 2,000 calories:

Breakfast: Four eggs, 300 calories, 28 grams of protein; two yogurts, 260 calories, 30 grams of protein

Lunch: Healthy Choice steamer frozen meal, plus ¼ pound sliced turkey, 365 calories, 44 grams protein

4:00 p.m. Shake: 1.5 shakes (3 scoops), 165 calories, 31 grams protein

Evening meal: 900 calories, 30 grams protein

Total: 1,990 calories, 163 grams protein

Shorter men may need to adjust this downward.

Similarly, shorter women, who may be overweight in the 130s or 140s, may have to trim the recommended female diet down as well. The nice thing about a standardized diet for 75 percent of the day is that it makes it easy to try something for a while and then allows for adjustments if results are not forthcoming.

Weekly Schedule

Most diet books would now present to you a complex weekly schedule of what to eat when. Not this one. **Remember you are eating the same food every day.** There will come a time, when you maintain, where you can perhaps scale The Boring Diet back to breakfast only.

There is no schedule, because there is nothing to schedule. Every day, you eat boring, until the cycle of addiction is broken.

Daily Weighing

Numerous studies have shown that daily weighing is beneficial. I recommend taking a daily weight in the morning and recording it. Ignore short-term trends, but over the long-term it will keep you motivated and accountable.

Link: https://tinyurl.com/dailyweigh

How It Works

What I've shared above is an idealized menu. The details could change, but as long as the calorie and protein targets are hit, it should work. So how exactly does it work? The animal appetite is stimulated by three primary motivations:

- Tasty combinations of carbohydrates and fat, especially with sugar, or just sugar by itself. This is why the low-carb diets work well, at least as long as people can stick to them.

- Instant gratification: It would much prefer an Oreo cookie now than a fantastic gourmet dessert later in the week.

- Variety: It loses motivation and gets bored if the same foods are offered repeatedly.

The Boring Diet attacks all three of these areas. Instead of reducing calories on the Standard

American Diet, full of temptations that will stimulate hunger, it voluntarily gives up much of the pleasure of food in advance, to avoid the pain of hunger later. It is a permanent lifestyle change such that food must occupy a smaller share of your mind.

Summary

I realize I've presented the plan a bit out of order procedurally, even if arranged logically in terms of ideas. So here's a quick summary of The Boring Diet:

1. Choose a monotonous menu of boring foods that puts you in a calorie deficit while providing lots of protein.

2. Take particularly pleasurable foods off the menu entirely.

3. When hungry, eat a boring, unprocessed snack: bananas, carrots, apples, or turkey slices. Eat these as necessary to train the animal instincts to only ask for food when nutritionally necessary, not for short-term hits of pleasure. Find pleasure in other daily activities that are not harmful to your body.

4. Have a protein shake at 4:00 p.m. every day.

5. Eat a moderate evening meal with a large portion of lean meat when possible.

6. If hungry, see #3.

7. Weigh yourself daily, in the morning, to keep yourself honest and motivated.

That's It?

This is a short book and a simple plan. I am a busy person, and so are you, so I didn't fluff out this book with a bunch of anecdotes and dramatic narratives. I tried to stick to the facts and save both of us time.

Though short and to the point, it is based on the latest research into our eating behavior, and I believe it represents the easiest and most realistic way for people to experience true weight loss and maintenance. It's not necessarily easy, and to be sure there will be some psychological adjustment.

For me, I had to stop using food as a psychological crutch to get through the day. As human beings with flesh-and-blood bodies that are every bit a part of who we are as our spirit, we need pleasure as part of our lives. The key, and in my view a key struggle of our spiritual life, is to receive these pleasures in legitimate ways that do not hurt us in the long run. Christians of a vintage era would call these the "lawful pleasures."

Food is a lawful pleasure, as long as it is not consumed in excess. Sex is a lawful pleasure, but nearly all cultures place strict limits around it because of its power. Both of these animal pleasures are necessary and normal, but easy to abuse. If food is a pleasure that has turned gluttonous, a part of the adjustment process of The Boring Diet is to give space for new pleasures to fill the void formerly provided by food.

New pleasures might include reading or intellectual pursuits, music, exercise, sewing, woodworking, or any sort of hobby where pleasure is balanced with effort such that gluttony is difficult. One's life must change from a food-centric pursuit of pleasure to generating pleasure from a variety of healthy activities.

Pleasure is not the enemy, but pleasure out of balance with what is good for us in the long-term is harmful. And frankly, pleasure that we know is bad for us will diminish our self-respect. Without self-respect, all of our experience of pleasure will be diminished. There is an ugly cycle of addiction, where indulging in too much pleasure makes people feel bad about themselves, which means they need even more pleasure to feel good again.

Successfully changing one's relationship with food–making it "boring" for the most part–ultimately increases our pleasure in life as we fulfill God's design for our bodies. When we fulfill God's design in any area of our life, we are naturally happier and more at peace. Or as the supermodel and practical philosopher Kate Moss put it, "Nothing tastes as good as being thin feels." This is especially true with our bodies because we are physical creatures, and the discipline to crucify our flesh and make it obey us is a sign of a spiritual tranquility underneath.

Getting Real About Junk Food

This is a chapter I decided to write just as the book was finishing up. It occurred to me that a lot of diet books have been sold, and while most of them work because of their common exclusion of ultra-processed junk food, the reality is that very few of the people who read the book lose any significant weight. I'm not sure if there's anything a writer can do to avoid that, but I'm going to try.

Many of my readers will have read this far and agree with what I have to say. Some may feel hopeful about a new approach that might work, and feel that sense of excitement we all feel when new plans have not yielded to the daily grind of execution on those same plans. It will seem as if anything is possible, but this feeling is fleeting.

But, some of those same people, perhaps you, will have quietly dismissed my recommendation to throw junk food in the trash and never allow it to return to one's personal environment again. The Boring Diet sounds great and all that, but I don't *really* have to do something as extreme as throwing a bunch of perfectly good food away, surely?

I suppose it depends on your true intention. Are you here to read a book and get some information to feel hopeful for a few weeks, or to take action and get results? One of the core ideas of The Boring Diet is that food addiction is **exactly like** any kind of substance addiction.

No one would argue that an alcoholic should keep some liquor around "just in case" or that to remove the immediate temptation would somehow be wasteful or unnecessary. Similarly, people who shoot heroin don't need to keep a stash around. Those with behavioral addictions, like sex or gambling problems, don't need to keep triggers around that are associated with the compulsive behavior.

Being at an unhealthy weight is almost always a symptom of a substance abuse problem—only here, the substance happens to be food. But not just any food. It is crap, processed foods like Oreos, Nutter Butters, ice cream, sodas, candy, potato chips, and the like. These serve no legitimate purpose for someone trying to get control of their eating habits, any more than alcohol in the house serves a purpose for the recovering alcoholic.

Junk food comes in all kinds of varieties that defy explanation as to why they're so appealing. Remember our rat experimenters, who tried all sorts of macronutrient combinations in rat chow without success in getting the rats to significantly overeat. Western supermarket food, however, did the trick in no time.

Few appreciate how competitive the packaged food industry is. The box of cereal, or the tray of cookies, is the most profitable item in a grocery store. A few pennies of raw materials are sold for several dollars, leaving lots of money left over for advertising and research into making the products as addictive as possible.

Every year, hundreds of new junk food products are launched. Most fail, so the ones that survive are the result of a ruthless Darwinian process where only the most addictive survive. Food companies spend billions employing food scientists and engineers to make their products more desirable.

I took a food engineering class in college, and one assignment was to use integral calculus to optimize the crunch of a tortilla chip. We had a device that would crush the chips with a little metal rod, hooked to a computer, and the computer would graph the force required to move through the chip over time. They knew, from many years of studies, the type of "crunch profile" that consumers desired and would result in the most addictive use pattern with their products.

Similarly, the soda industry knows about the "bliss point," that is the optimal amount of sugar and sweetness to maximize compulsive consumption. They also know that more sugar is inherently addictive, so they spike their products with phosphoric acid that balances the sweet on our taste buds. This is all to push the amount of sugar we tolerate at the "bliss point" even higher, increase the sugar rush, induce a sugar crash so we drink more, and enhance the pleasure of the product. This is why soda has so much more sugar than say iced tea or coffee. Without these chemical modifications to trick us into drinking more sugar, we would spit soda out of our mouth for being too sickly sweet.

These people don't play. They own multi-billion-dollar businesses selling legal addictive substances, and your animal appetites are no match for the temptation of having them in close proximity. If this weren't true, why has weight always been a struggle? If you could eat this stuff in moderation, why haven't you done it already?

The three biggest Internet companies, Google, Facebook, and Amazon, are obsessed with the speed of their websites. They have internal research showing how much money they lose for each millisecond longer it takes for their site to load. Just a little bit of waiting or lagging and users get frustrated, turning their attention to other distractions, and, in turn, not clicking on ads. Just as these companies want to decrease the friction in your consuming ads on their platforms, to lose weight we must increase the friction of eating junk food while decreasing the friction of eating boring foods.

I think a common thread behind many diet failures is that there is an eagerness to do new things, like eat more meat, but an unwillingness to eliminate behaviors that primarily caused the problem. It's as if the junk food becomes a sort of "my precious"–like the Gollum character in *Lord of the Rings*–that is protected at all costs from any plan of action to eliminate the temptation.

This, again, is the animal instinct, the lower part of our nature, attempting to masquerade as the true self. It will use fallacious arguments all day to hold on to its "precious." I encourage you to separate your conception of your true self from these lies, and to use the human part of your brain to overcome your animal desires. This is the essence of what it means to be human, and each and every one of us can do it. If you haven't taken action yet to eliminate these foods, do it now. Do it while you have the will to do so and before you change your mind. Our feelings follow our actions, and our actions are the only things we really control, so take massive action now and let your feelings take care of themselves later.

Only when these hunger-stimulating temptations are removed can The Boring Diet do its work.

Details, Questions, Objections

The Boring Diet is simple, but it is not necessarily easy. The diet brings one face-to-face with the reality that hunger is negotiable. It's situational and it changes based on the foods we offer it. If we reduce the overall pleasure of eating and offer the animal appetite simple foods when it claims to be hungry, we will find hunger much reduced.

However, difficulties will inevitably come up when attempting such a drastic dietary change. In no particular order, I'll address some particular challenges and objections in this chapter.

Nutrition

Some will dismiss this approach to diet because it is monotonous, and think that it must not have enough variety to provide all of the vitamins and nutrition we need. My answer to that is that The Boring Diet generally isn't replacing kale salads tossed with cashews, extra virgin olive oil, apple cider vinegar, and fresh-grilled wild salmon. What the diet does is replace really bad food choices, say a fast food lunch, with something relatively bland and nutritious.

We start the day with high quality, highly bioavailable, easy-to-prepare, and inexpensive animal protein in the form of eggs and dairy, both of which are loaded with essential vitamins.

The midday frozen meal, while perhaps boring, is quite nutritious. The types of Healthy Choice or Lean Cuisine type meals I am recommending are usually loaded with lean meat and vegetables, and rotating among three to four varieties mixes up the nutrition from day-to-day. The freezing process locks in all of the goodness of fresh vegetables, without preservatives, and so provides good sources of vitamins and other dietary necessities. The afternoon protein shake uses the most bioavailable form of protein, whey, while addressing the most common dietary deficiency even among those who overeat in general.

For the evening meal The Boring Diet allows for unlimited variety, at least when it comes to nutritious food. Last time I checked, pizza, bread, candy, chips, and soda were not an essential part of anyone's nutrition. The boring snacks provided to stave off hunger are likewise whole, nutritious foods–fruits, vegetables, and lean protein. The Boring Diet is the opposite of processed, artificial nutrition. It is more like the limited but adequate variety of nutritious, but not terribly exciting, foods our ancestors had access to before the junk food industry made most people fat.

Breakfast Alternatives

The monotonous, high-protein daily breakfast is the heart of The Boring Diet. One of my early readers for this book asked about what to do when someone has an allergy or aversion to eggs or dairy.

Personally, I don't like eggs, and I did not use eggs for my monotonous breakfasts. I include them here because they are such a high-protein, nutritionally-dense food, but I find the sulfur taste unbearable, and I have not yet disciplined myself to eat them. A good friend of mine eats six eggs a day, along with a low-carbohydrate diet he actually sticks to most of the time, and his blood test results have been phenomenal. But what to do for those of us who don't like or can't eat eggs?

In this section, I'll list some alternatives that still meet our bland and high-protein morning requirements. However, to maximize the effectiveness of the diet, I do not recommend mixing and matching. **Pick one breakfast and stick to it.** Breakfast, because it is not typically a social meal, is your one big opportunity to hit 100 percent adherence to the program, and it sets the tone for the rest of the day. The more you treat meals like a menu instead of boring nutrition, the less effective the neurocognitive retraining will be.

The blogger Scott Alexander of SlateStarCodex.com reviewed *The Hungry Brain* and identified a food product that perfectly encapsulates the teaching of the book. He recommends buying MealSquares (MealSquares.com), which are ready-to-eat, bland, 400-calorie, high-protein, nutritionally complete baked "muffins." Don't get too excited; there's a reason I put "muffins" in scare quotes. I have tried them, and I can report that they are as advertised: just plain nutrition. They are quite dry, which is good, because they expand in the stomach, so you will want to eat them with plenty of water. One MealSquare with water (400 calories, 20 grams of protein) is probably perfect for most women on The Boring Diet, with perhaps the addition of a low-sugar Greek yogurt (an additional 130 calories, 15 grams of protein). Men would likely want to add a glass of whole milk (150 calories, 8 grams protein) and a low-sugar Greek yogurt.

MealSquares are excellent for those with an aversion to eggs, but they do contain eggs. For those with an egg allergy, I recommend doing a double serving, for women, or triple serving, for men, of a low-sugar Greek yogurt. This may be mixed with ½ cup of the original Ezekial 4:9 unsweetened, sprouted grain cereal (190 calories, 8 grams protein). You guessed it; it doesn't taste that exciting, but it is very crunchy and takes quite a while to eat. Be sure to measure the cereal, as it is easy to overdo.

For those with a dairy allergy, the intake of eggs can be scaled up to four a day for women or five to six a day for men. If that's too many, stick to the original egg recommendation and add ¼ pound of lean deli ham, which you can sauté in a nonstick skillet with cooking spray or make into an omelet with the eggs.

If making an omelet, you can add all the non-starchy vegetables you want.

Any of these alternatives will get you in the same zone of calories and protein as the original egg and yogurt recommendation.

Adherence

I almost don't want to write this section, because I don't want to encourage the addictive overeating voice with a way to rationalize not sticking to the plan. However, I should admit that I still lost weight without following this plan perfectly.

So don't quit because you mess up one time. We want to avoid black-and-white thinking. There is an error in thinking that people get into that psychologists call the "what the hell" effect. If we mess up a little bit on a plan, there is a temptation to just say "what the hell, I messed it up" and then use that opportunity to binge eat.

It's certainly hard to eat just one cookie, but eating one cookie isn't going to change the outcome of The Boring Diet. On the other hand, eating ten cookies every day will mess up fat loss efforts, especially if eating the first cookie serves to justify the rest.

So the ideal is to resist the first temptation to avoid the second. But in no case should we get into all-or-nothing thinking and totally abandon the plan because we make a mistake or two.

The Boring Diet is a double-barreled approach to fat loss. It eliminates addictive foods and provides a monotony of healthy foods that should repair the body's signaling mechanisms and cause it to spontaneously be less hungry even while eating fewer calories.

Perfect adherence is not necessary for it to work, especially at first. But, knowing we will not be perfect is not an excuse to be imperfect right now.

There is a similar paradox at the heart of the Christian theology of sin. It says we have the power to overcome any one temptation, that we literally never face a situation where we are helpless to give in. On the other hand, it recognizes that some failures, in the aggregate, are inevitable and provides grace for those situations.

Treat your fat loss efforts the same way. Be ruthlessly zealous when dealing with any one temptation, the one that's right in front of you right now, but don't be carried away by a sense of failure if you mess up. The Boring Diet can work with a lot of mistakes.

If you follow the plan of eating the same monotonous, healthy menu, it should be easy to "reset" the next day whenever there's a mess-up. Don't wallow in failure; pick yourself up and start again. Your inner animal instinct can be vicious. If allowed, it will gladly use despair, perfectionism, and bitterness as excuses for re-indulging in addictive behaviors.

Women & Smaller Men

This is another section I almost didn't want to include. We live in a hyper-sensitive, overly-politicized environment, and even things like obvious biological facts can be seen as controversial. But I respect you as my reader, and I believe I have to share all of the relevant facts. One set of important facts involves the average differences between men and women when it comes to weight loss efforts.

Smaller people can't eat as much without gaining fat, and women cannot eat as much as men at the same height and weight. Men, due to the effects of testosterone, have higher muscle mass, are on average larger, with a higher metabolism and a higher red blood cell count. As a result, men burn more calories just as part of normal life than women do. In general, women need significantly fewer calories than men to maintain the same weight, and must eat fewer calories to lose weight. This, of course, would not apply to elite female athletes, who may eat more than sedentary men just to maintain weight and avoid losing critical muscle mass.

Some scientists have started to describe our food environment as **obesogenic**–it literally creates obesity. Let's take just one example, the big temptation of eating out at a restaurant. Portions have gotten enormous. Let's say a portion at a restaurant is 500 calories larger than what someone would serve themselves at home. For a typical man with a calorie maintenance need of 2500 calories, this is much easier to absorb than the typical woman with a daily calorie maintenance need of 2000 calories. Restaurants serve the same huge portion to everyone, but women pay a bigger consequence for indulging.

Women have to adopt a mindset of realism about how much food is appropriate for their smaller bodies (or the smaller body they aspire to). This is one area where seeking equality with men, in terms of quantity of food eaten, can only end with worse outcomes for women. At restaurants in particular, women must pay attention to calorie counts much more than men.

Because men must eat more to maintain weight, a man can cut more calories more easily and still lose weight. A man on a diet might eat as much as an overweight woman maintaining her weight. This can seem unfair, if only because overeating has become such a central part of our culture. Women do live longer than men, so the total amount of food consumed in a lifetime might be about the same.

Public health authorities already make an important distinction between men and women in one particular area: alcohol intake recommendations. Women are advised to drink about half as much as men because their bodies, with smaller livers, cannot process it as efficiently. With alcohol, it's life and death, because a woman who binge drinks like a typical partying man may accidentally kill herself by alcohol poisoning.

Just as most women accept that they cannot drink like a man, women who wish to be healthy and thin must accept they cannot eat like a man either. The consequences may be slower to take effect, but they are every bit as devastating in the long run as overconsuming alcohol.

Smaller men must also accept that they may need to eat less than their larger peers.

Exercise

I have not mentioned exercise much in this book. This is on purpose. Fat loss is 80 percent diet, and no amount of exercise can undo the damage of sugar sodas, Chips Ahoy, or Doritos. However, this is not to say I do not value exercise at all.

The processed food companies, to protect their ability to sell harmful and addictive products, have for years funded research pushing the "calories in, calories out" simplistic model of weight loss. They desperately want to convince you that the problem isn't Coca-Cola being marketed to children, but rather you being lazy.

It seems to me that many overweight people, in no small part due to this propaganda, link exercise to weight loss quite strongly, much more strongly than research suggests is appropriate. This can result in a strange dynamic where people seek to "earn" the right to eat bad food, as long as they exercise.

Some of the fitness subcultures encourage this, with a "macho" attitude towards food, that somehow because they are so extreme in their workouts, they don't have to worry about what they eat, or as long as they eat "clean" with many paleo-approved junk food options.

This is probably true for someone like Michael Phelps, but your average fitness boot camp attendee is not an elite athlete. Those who don't watch diet become more muscled overweight people, certainly beneficial but not as much as some seem to think.

Unfortunately, while exercise is beneficial to health, it is not a substitute for fat loss. Overweight and obese people who are metabolically healthy are still 25 percent more likely to have adverse health events than those with normal weight.

Link: https://tinyurl.com/healthyobesity

The reality is that exercise, at best, helps us maintain weight. It has other profound benefits on psychology and is the most effective thing we can do to prevent depression and anxiety. It can even become a highly pleasurable hobby that can fill the hole left by abandoning junk food.

Nevertheless, and I've observed this firsthand, I think with some people exercise becomes a crutch to negotiate with themselves to get permission to overeat. The animal appetite will use any excuse to get what it wants. And while it would prefer not to exercise at all, it will gladly trade exercise if that enables it to continue eating junk food. It will use all of its wiles to trick your rational mind into justifying a pint of ice cream with 500 calories because you ran a mile and burned 100 calories earlier in the day. It would certainly rather have the ice cream by itself, but from its perspective it still scored a 400 calorie profit.

There is one form of exercise that is particularly beneficial to those wanting fat loss and should be prioritized. This is resistance exercise. While all weight loss involves a loss of fat and muscle, one of the reasons The Boring Diet includes a lot of protein is that it tends to minimize the loss of muscle, which is so critical to metabolism, health, and maintaining weight. Similarly, resistance exercise, or lifting weights, sends a signal to the body that it shouldn't allow too much muscle to be used for fuel, and it should burn fat instead.

Diet, almost alone, determines weight loss. Resistance exercise and protein intake determines the type of weight lost, and with both, fat loss is maximized.

To learn more about resistance exercise, I highly recommend the website StrongerLifts.com. It is full of completely free resources teaching anyone how to lift weights with barbells, including the critical full-body exercises of squats and deadlift. The emphasis of a systematic approach of increasing weight on the bar is particularly powerful.

The Valley of Fat Loss

If a person is overweight or obese, there are profound health benefits to losing and maintaining a loss of even ten pounds. Weight loss tends to be easy at first, and the benefits in terms of health, energy, mobility, and overall well-being are undeniable. Appearance-wise, going from obese to the upper end of normal weight is especially motivating. However, most will have difficulty going from the upper end of "normal" to optimally thin. Weight loss gets more difficult, and the rewards in terms of appearance and self-image are slower in coming.

"Normal" weight is, for most people, still overweight. The BMI guidelines are very generous, and while they may misclassify some extreme bodybuilders as overweight despite low body fat, for most people they tend to severely overestimate what weight is normal and healthy. One study in Italy–a country notably thinner than the United States–found that when body fat percentage rather than BMI was measured, there was a prevalence of overweight and obesity of about 85 percent for women and 69 percent for men.

Link: https://tinyurl.com/bmifatstudy

So if we start telling ourselves we're healthy once we reach a "normal" BMI, we will lose motivation to continue the journey. Instead, we should measure body fat. The US Navy developed a method for estimating body fat using body measurements that is more accurate than traditional caliper techniques and is definitely more useful than BMI. Since weight is not used in the formula, but rather direct body measurements (including adjusting for frame size) it avoids the inaccuracies of BMI. There is an online calculator here for the method:

Link: https://tinyurl.com/navybodyfat

Then compare your body fat percentage to the body fat ranges recommended by the American Council on Exercise:

Table 6.14
General Body-fat Percentage Categories

Classification	Women (% fat)	Men (% fat)
Essential fat	10 - 13%	2 - 5%
Athletes	14 - 20%	6 - 13%
Fitness	21 - 24 %	14 - 17%
Average	25 - 31%	18 - 24%
Obese	32% and higher	25% and higher

We want to aim for "fitness" or "athlete" for the best effects on health. I recommend measuring yourself weekly and computing your body fat percentage with the calculator linked above, in addition to daily weighing. Ultimately, we want fat loss, and healthy body fat levels, and our weight is only an imperfect directional indicator.

One of the big problems, and I'm being real here, is that we don't really care about our health as much as we might think we do. What we really care about is how we look, and I don't think there's anything necessarily wrong with that. Since what looks good is also what's healthy, in general, it's good we have some practical motivation in the short-term to overcome the temptations of junk food surrounding us.

The problem is that while the health benefits continue to go up with each pound lost, the effect on our appearance tends to stall out after some big initial gains. We seem to have three basic categories mentally—we see other people, and ourselves, as either obese, average/overweight, or fit. There's a huge benefit health-wise and appearance-wise going from obese to merely overweight. The journey from average/overweight to fit, however, is much longer and tougher, and the payoff in appearance and self-image doesn't come until almost the very end.

A study out of the University of Texas from 2012 validates this distortion in our perceptions, where perceived appearance tends to "flatline" along the vast region between average and fit. In this study, women had their body fat percentage directly measured via DEXA scans, and an anonymized outline of their body shapes from the DEXA scan were shown to volunteers, male and female, to rate their attractiveness:

Link: https://tinyurl.com/dexastudy

The chart below shows the relationship between body fat percentage and perceived attractiveness:

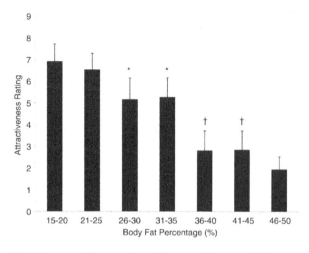

Fig. 4. Mean attractiveness ratings (with standard deviation) for images in each BF% category. All categories are significantly different than each other ($p<.01$, $N=127$) except between 26%–30% and 31%–35% (notated by *, $p>.05$) and between 36%–40% and 41%–45% (notated by †, $p>.05$).

At first, dropping from 36 to 40 percent body fat results in a huge improvement in perceived attractiveness. As body fat dropped from 35 percent to 26 percent, however, perceived appearance did not go up at all. A 9 percent drop in body fat in this zone would bring profound health improvements, but little encouragement in terms of self-image. While this study involves women, no doubt the same would hold true of men, relatively speaking–men, of course, require lower body fat than women to look good.

I think this is perhaps why weight loss efforts stall out. We aren't as rational about our health as we think we are, and our real motivation, much of the time, is appearance. Once the easy wins are out of the way by moving from obese to merely overweight or average, people lose motivation, and the allure of former lusts are too enticing to resist.

This also explains why gaining weight from year to year is so easy. Once someone lets themselves go, say after marriage or having children, and moves out of the fit range, there is a lot of weight that can be gained in the overweight category without any significant negative impact on the appearance. No one consciously chooses to be obese; they get there one step at a time responding to incentives and costs immediately in front of them.

The only way to break this cycle is to realize that our perceptions are messed up relative to the benefits to our health. To reach fitness, continued efforts require an iron resolve to keep the vision firmly locked on the goal. Once you arrive there, it will be worth it, but it will require months of adherence to a weight-loss plan without huge payoffs in how you look until almost the very end. And when you really think about it, a goal of true fitness is much more motivating than just becoming less overweight.

In the business world, author Jim Collins calls this the Big Hairy Audacious Goal – or BHAG. Human beings are motivated by big goals more than smaller ones. If you set a goal of getting your body fat percentage in the fitness or athletic range, which would result, for example, of looking good at the beach, you may find you are much more willing to work for that goal than a more modest goal of losing 10% of your body weight, which is the standard medical advice for those who need to lose weight. While it may be more achievable theoretically, it may not be in practice.

One other benefit of pushing into the true fitness range is that maintaining weight becomes much more motivating. Instead of weight gain resulting in you becoming slightly pudgier, which might not be noticeable, any significant fat gains will immediately start impacting your perceived appearance. For example, just a few pounds of fat on a man, right around the waist, is necessary to turn a fit bod into a dad bod. But if you're sporting the dad bod already, a slightly bigger dad bod doesn't feel so bad, especially when food is always so compelling right now.

With The Boring Diet, you don't have to be hungry, just bored with your food. As weight loss slows, as it inevitably will, more action may have to be taken to continue the journey. This may mean eliminating more forbidden foods, or cracking down on rogue snacking or cheat meals. This may mean eliminating the non-bread starchy carbohydrates, like potatoes or rice, or other foods you like too much, entirely. It's tough, I know it's tough, but only you can decide if it's worth it.

My only promise is that with The Boring Diet, you can do it mostly without the torment of hunger. The decision to trade the short-term pleasure of indulging in bad food for the long-term pleasure of health, appearance, and energy is yours alone to make.

What if I'm Already Fit

If you're already at a fit and healthy weight, I would bet you fall into one of three categories:

1. Exceptional genetics: You eat a Standard American Diet, yet you've never gained significant weight.

2. Fit Heritage: You grew up in a home or around peers where self-restraint with food was part of your culture.

3. Fit Self-Made: Like me, you struggled with weight in the past, but made a major lifestyle and worldview change to become fit.

If you're in this first group, consider yourself lucky, but also warned. With 80+ percent of the population destined to eventually be overweight or obese, don't be overconfident that you will continue to be the exception. As I've gotten older, most of my formerly naturally-skinny friends who ate whatever they wanted are starting to get pudgy. Since they're not doing weight training or hard labor either, the natural loss of muscle with age has also set in. "Skinny fat" is not a good look.

Perhaps the biggest tragedy I see is families with skinny parents and fat kids. Both parents have a genetic gift, or perhaps the cultural-based self control of Group 2 above, but somehow either the genes or the culture did not get passed to the kids. The parents continue to serve crap food to the family, or have crap food generally available in the house, and the kids get fat.

If you are the rare person who can eat whatever, or be around junk food and eat it moderately, and not gain weight, odds are your kids, at least not all of them, will not be that way. The food engineers at Frito-Lay and Coca-Cola have other plans for your children. Absent intervention to counter the obesity culture around your children, they will likely also succumb. At minimum, children should be required to ask before eating any snack other than whole fruits and vegetables, and parents should restrict them to reasonable portions. Sweets in particular must be subject to parental approval before they are consumed.

For the third group, or those reading this book who want to be in the third group, consider how self-made fitness is really the best and most reliable form of fitness. Genetics and culture can only get you so far, and if our society continues down the path it's on, it will get harder and harder to be fit on accident. If our approach is deliberate, based on an intentional desire to be different than the society around us, we are much more likely to succeed in maintaining lost weight and "changing our family tree."

I believe no small part of my motivation to lose and keep off extra fat was because I did not want my children to experience the same thing I did. Children learn from example more than instruction, and I simply knew there was no way my vision for them was compatible with my continuing to abuse my body with junk food.

Artificial & Natural Low-Calorie Sweeteners

This was discussed briefly earlier in the book explaining why diet drinks are not an acceptable substitute for conventional sodas. In theory, artificial sweeteners should be safe. In practice, for reasons no one understands, they're not. People who consume them in drinks seem to have the same or worse health problems as those who drink sugar-sweetened beverages.

The cause of the problems may not the chemicals themselves. No one has proposed a plausible way for them to harm humans chemically, and extended experiments with animals has shown harmlessness at extremely high doses. The issue is probably due to the stimulation of the sweetness itself. One theory is that the body doesn't like being tricked, and ramps up hunger big-time later in the day when it knows it's been fooled by sweet flavor followed by zero calories.

There are a few natural low-calorie sweeteners in common use today, notably stevia, monk fruit extract, and various sugar alcohols. If the sweet-but-no-calories issue is what's driving the problem with artificial sweeteners, that would hold true for natural low-calorie sweeteners too.

At the same time, I would think the damage done from a natural substance would be less than that from an artificial one. The chemical reasons for this are complex, but in summary I think natural substances are generally safer because all organic life forms use a limited set of chemical pathways, producing chemical patterns that other life forms are more adept at processing. We are not so good at processing chemicals exclusively derived from lab synthesis rather than natural processes. That's my guess, anyway.

The best practice is to avoid all low-calorie sweeteners. However, this is not practical, at least for me. So my rule is that I never drink anything sweetened, artificial or not, except a tiny bit of sugar in my morning coffee. I'm okay, however, with using stevia, monk fruit, or other natural low-calorie sweeteners to enhance my protein intake. So I eat the stuff in protein bars, powders, etc.

I feel like this is less harmful than a diet drink because the sweet flavor is accompanied by some calories, just different calories, typically derived from protein and fat. Hopefully this satisfies the body's expectation of nutrition with sweet flavor, and it doesn't overreact later with hunger. So far this has been my experience. I also chew xylitol-based gum with no ill effect, and this is great for oral health.

One other practice I'm very skeptical of is the use of natural sweeteners like stevia or sugar alcohols to make what paleo enthusiasts call "fat bombs." Typically made with nut flours and coconut oil, perhaps with unsweetened cocoa, these are meant to satisfy a dessert craving for those on a strict paleo diet. All of the ingredients are low carb, but all are also heavily processed relative to ancestral diets.

We know from the neuroscience that the taste of sweetness combined with fat is very addictive and palatable. It's possible that even a natural low-calorie sweetener would provide the hedonistic payoff one might get from conventional candy. Remember what makes us hungry is food we like too much, not carbs per-se. So, my rule is that these sweeteners, if used, must be accompanied with significant protein (which usually also degrades the taste, in the case of protein powders and bars), not used to create fatty, sweet desserts that check a low carb box.

If you're able to avoid both natural and artificial low-calorie sweeteners, good for you. I'm just sharing a reasonable compromise that has worked for me.

Final Thoughts

As I'm rushing this book to press in December 2019, I came across another study that puts some surprising numbers on the obesity crisis. The best estimates now show that 91 percent of American adults and 69 percent of children are overweight. This is an unbelievable tragedy and health crisis.

Link: https://tinyurl.com/overfatstudy

Strangely, we are now a society where to be normal requires appearing extreme. By any standard, it's the society around us that is extreme.

If you look at old vintage photos of American life, hardly anyone was overweight. Something profound has changed in our society, and to be "normal" in the good sense requires being different. As Dave Ramsey says regarding finances: "if you want to live like no one else, you have to live like no one else."

I will say that it gets easier over time. I do not currently follow The Boring Diet to nearly the same level as when I was trying to lose weight. After a few years of maintaining, it seems the body settles in to the new normal and accepts the new thermostat setting for weight.

I do still follow a few general rules. I eat a small variety of relatively boring, healthy, high-protein breakfasts. I try to avoid more than one piece of bread a day. I fill up on meat and other proteins instead of starch. And the starches I do eat are relatively unprocessed. I still abstain from soda, as my old addiction, Coca-Cola, remains as enticing as ever. The few times I've had one since quitting: let's just say I understand why it's so tempting. There is something magical about the effervescence of the flavor notes, and I simply like it too much to have it at all.

I eat the occasional dessert, as do my children. It's just that we do it at a frequency much more akin to how it was done in the past – when great-grandma baked the occasional sweet – than how it's done today with the ubiquity of ready-made desserts. We have dessert no more than once a day, and not every day. When my clothes start to get a little tight, I follow Grandma's advice and cut the starches and sweets for a bit. If necessary, I go back to The Boring Diet for a few days. To me, that doesn't seem extreme. What's extreme from my new vantage point is trading my health for the momentary and fading pleasure of junk food.

Normal, healthy weight is very doable. It was doable 100 years ago, when most people did it, and it is doable today. Only you can decide if you are willing to make the journey. If you do, you have my encouragement as you seek to change your family tree as well.

Made in the USA
Monee, IL
08 March 2020